NEUROFEEDBA CK THERAPY

A Comprehensive Guide To Exploring Brain Function, Treatment Principles Integrative Approaches, Ethical Insights, And Future Horizons For Healing And Growth

WILFREDO CARSON

INTRODUCTION

Neurofeedback treatment is a cutting-edge therapeutic intervention that has been recognized for its ability to treat a wide range of neurological and psychiatric problems.

This method entails real-time monitoring of brain activity and providing feedback to the user to facilitate self-regulation of brain function. Neurofeedback is founded on an understanding of the brain's ability to adapt and restructure itself, often known as neuroplasticity. This introduction will look at the history of neurofeedback therapy, the scientific concepts that underpin its success, its various applications, and the overall scope and aim of this book.

1.1 What is neurofeedback therapy?

Neurofeedback therapy, also known as EEG biofeedback or neurotherapy, is a non-invasive method for regulating brain function by giving individuals real-time data on their brainwave patterns. This procedure is placing sensors on the scalp to monitor electrical activity in the brain, specifically the electroencephalogram (EEG). Individuals can learn to self-regulate their brain activity by providing this information visually or auditorily, resulting in more balanced and efficient functioning. The main principle is founded on the idea that the brain can learn and adapt and that by providing feedback, humans may deliberately control and optimize brain function.

1.2 Historical Development of Neurofeedback

The history of neurofeedback may be traced back to the mid-twentieth century when researchers began investigating the link between brainwave patterns and different mental and emotional states. The initial focus was on understanding the brain's electrical activity and its relationship to disorders like epilepsy. Notably, in the 1960s and 1970s, pioneers such as Dr. Barry Sterman began testing operant conditioning of brainwaves to regulate epileptic seizures. Over the years, technological improvements have played a critical role in improving neurofeedback equipment and techniques, allowing for more precise and customized interventions. Neurofeedback has progressed from its early experimental stages to its current status as a well-established treatment modality with applications for a wide spectrum of neurological and psychological disorders.

1.3 The Science of Neurofeedback.

The science of neurofeedback therapy is based on an understanding of brainwave patterns and how they relate to different mental states. The brain generates electrical activity in the form of oscillating waves that fall into certain frequency ranges such as delta, theta, alpha, beta, and gamma. Each of these bands is linked to distinct cognitive and emotional functions. Neurofeedback is based on assessing an individual's unique brainwave patterns and detecting any dysregulation or imbalance. Individuals can learn to modify their brainwave activity by providing real-time feedback, which typically takes the form of visual or aural cues. This process is based on the concepts of operant conditioning, in which the brain is rewarded for producing desired patterns and pushed to self-regulate towards a more optimal condition. Neuroplasticity research supports the premise that the brain can adapt and restructure itself in response to experiences and feedback, making neurofeedback an effective technique for improving brain function.

1.4 Applications for Neurofeedback Therapy

Neurofeedback therapy has shown promise in treating a variety of neurological and psychological problems. One widely used application is the therapy of attention-deficit/hyperactivity disorder (ADHD). Neurofeedback training has been shown to treat ADHD symptoms by teaching people how to manage their attention and focus.

Neurofeedback has also shown potential in treating anxiety and mood disorders because it allows people to change their brainwave patterns associated with stress and emotional regulation. Additionally, neurofeedback has been used in the rehabilitation of traumatic brain injuries, assisting individuals in recovering cognitive function and improving general well-being. Beyond therapeutic applications, neurofeedback has grown in popularity as a peak performance training tool for athletes, musicians, and professionals looking to improve their cognitive talents and performance.

1.5 Scope and Purpose of The Book

The goal of this book is to provide a thorough examination of neurofeedback therapy, including its historical roots, the scientific foundations that underpin its effectiveness, its various uses, and possible future advances. This book aims to be a beneficial resource for clinicians, researchers, and anybody interested in learning more about neurofeedback by providing an in-depth examination and synthesis of existing information. By digging into the complexities of neurofeedback, readers will gain insight into its theoretical foundations, practical applications, and the ever-changing environment of this dynamic discipline. Finally, the goal of this book is to help spread knowledge and promote a broader appreciation for the potential of neurofeedback as a therapeutic intervention in the fields of mental health, neurorehabilitation, and human performance optimization.

CHAPTER 1
UNDERSTANDING THE BRAIN

<u>Anatomy and Function of the Brain</u>

The human brain, a tremendously complex organ, acts as the nervous system's fundamental command center, orchestrating different physical systems and cognitive processes. The brain, which has billions of neurons coupled by trillions of synapses, is organized into separate regions, each responsible for a certain function. The cerebral cortex, for example, is responsible for sensory perception, motor control, and higher cognitive skills, whereas the limbic system is involved in emotions and memory. Deep within the brain, regions such as the hippocampus and amygdala help with learning and emotional regulation.

A thorough understanding of the brain's structure is required to investigate neurofeedback therapy since it allows doctors to identify target areas for intervention.

Brainwave Patterns and Frequency

Brainwaves are rhythmic patterns of electrical activity in the brain that can be recorded with electroencephalography (EEG).

These brainwaves are divided into frequency bands, each of which corresponds to a unique state of awareness and cognitive function. Delta waves, which occur at the lowest frequencies (0.5 to 4 Hz), are associated with profound sleep and recovery. Theta waves (4 to 8 Hz) are common during light sleep and meditation. Alpha waves (8 to 13 Hz) are connected with comfortable wakefulness, whereas beta waves (13 to 30 Hz) represent active, focused thinking. Gamma waves (30 to 40 Hz and above) are linked to higher cognitive processes. Neurofeedback therapy seeks to control these brainwave patterns, promoting desired states and alleviating symptoms associated with dysregulation.

Neuroplasticity and its role in neurofeedback.

Neuroplasticity, a basic feature of the brain, refers to its ability to restructure and adapt in response to experience, learning, and injury. This dynamic process causes structural and functional changes in neural connections, allowing the brain to improve its functioning.

Neurofeedback therapy uses neuroplasticity to provide real-time information on brain activity, allowing people to learn how to self-regulate and change their neural networks. When people practice neurofeedback, the brain establishes new synaptic connections, strengthening beneficial patterns and decreasing maladaptive ones. Understanding the principles of neuroplasticity is critical for developing effective neurofeedback protocols customized to specific cognitive or emotional difficulties.

The Relationship Between Brain Function and Mental Health

Neurofeedback therapy is based on the complex relationship between brain function and mental wellness. Many mental health illnesses, such as anxiety, depression, attention-deficit/hyperactivity disorder (ADHD), and post-traumatic stress disorder (PTSD), are linked to abnormal brain activity patterns.

Neurofeedback aims to address these dysregulations by teaching people to self-regulate their brain activity, resulting in a more stable and adaptive neural state. Neurofeedback has promise as a non-invasive treatment for a variety of mental health issues since it promotes ideal brainwave patterns and encourages neuroplastic changes. Understanding the complicated links between brain function and mental health is critical for adapting neurofeedback protocols to meet the unique needs of individuals and improve overall well-being.

CHAPTER 2
PRINCIPLES OF NEUROFEEDBACK THERAPY

Neurofeedback therapy, also known as EEG biofeedback, is a non-invasive therapeutic technique that tries to control and enhance brain function by delivering real-time data on neural activity. The core ideas of neurofeedback therapy are based on the idea that the brain may be educated to self-regulate and achieve greater equilibrium.

The procedure involves monitoring brainwave patterns using electroencephalogram (EEG) equipment and offering feedback to individuals, allowing them to learn how to deliberately adjust their brain activity.

This type of Neurotherapy is based on the concept of operant conditioning, which uses positive reinforcement to stimulate desirable changes in brain function.

How Does Neurofeedback Work?

Neurofeedback uses modern neuroimaging techniques, such as EEG, to record and evaluate the electrical activity generated by the brain. During a neurofeedback session, sensors are placed on the scalp to capture electrical impulses generated by various brain areas. These signals are subsequently processed in real-time, with feedback delivered to the individual via visual or audible cues. Individuals can learn to intentionally change their brainwave patterns by receiving continuous feedback. The brain's remarkable adaptability allows it to gradually modify its activity in response to this feedback. Self-regulation is thought to promote cognitive, emotional, and behavioral abilities.

<u>Types of Neurofeedback Approaches:</u>

There are various neurofeedback approaches, each with its methodology and application. Surface neurofeedback is one strategy that includes attaching sensors to the scalp to monitor surface-level brainwave activity.

This strategy is often used to treat ADHD, anxiety, and stress. In contrast, Z-Score neurofeedback uses statistical analysis to compare an individual's brainwave patterns to a normative database. This technique allows for more targeted treatment, focusing on specific departures from the norm. LORETA (Low-Resolution Electromagnetic Tomography) neurofeedback is a more advanced technology that offers three-dimensional data on brain activity, allowing for precise targeting of malfunctioning regions.

Electroencephalography (EEG) with neurofeedback:

The electroencephalogram (EEG) is an important tool in the execution of neurofeedback therapy. EEG detects the electrical activity of the brain by monitoring voltage fluctuations caused by ionic current flow within neurons. This non-invasive procedure involves applying electrodes to the scalp to record the electrical impulses produced by the brain. The EEG data is then examined to determine specific brainwave frequencies like delta, theta, alpha, beta, and gamma. These frequencies are connected with varying levels of consciousness, attentiveness, and arousal.

In neurofeedback therapy, the EEG is the key tool for monitoring and providing feedback on these brainwave patterns, allowing patients to achieve conscious control over their neural activity.

Neurofeedback therapy is based on operant training principles, with EEG technology providing real-time feedback to assist self-regulation of brain activity. Surface neurofeedback, Z-Score neurofeedback, and LORETA neurofeedback are three different forms of neurofeedback approaches that provide individualized treatments for a variety of neurological and psychological disorders. The Electroencephalogram (EEG) is important in neurofeedback therapy because it provides a complete understanding of brainwave patterns, allowing for tailored therapies.

The application of these ideas in neurofeedback therapy shows promise for improving cognitive, emotional, and behavioral well-being by leveraging the brain's natural plasticity and adaptability.

CHAPTER 3
THE NEUROFEEDBACK PROCESS

The Neurofeedback Process begins with the critical stages of Initial Assessment and Client Evaluation. This phase is critical for determining the individual's unique neurophysiological profile and adapting the neurofeedback intervention accordingly. QEEG (Quantitative Electroencephalography) Mapping is a sophisticated method used in this examination to provide a thorough analysis of the brain's electrical activity. This approach identifies abnormal brainwave patterns and irregularities, providing significant insights into potential regions of dysregulation. Concurrently, professional interviews and a thorough examination of the client's past provide context for their psychological and neurological landscapes.

This multidimensional method ensures a comprehensive understanding of the individual's current state, which guides the next steps in the neurofeedback process.

Once the Initial Assessment is completed, the next step is to establish Treatment Goals. This critical phase requires coordination between the neurofeedback practitioner and the client to develop specific and quantifiable goals. These objectives serve as benchmarks for assessing the efficacy of the neurofeedback intervention over time. Importantly, they address the individual's specific concerns, whether they are related to cognitive function, emotional well-being, or behavioral challenges. The development of exact treatment goals improves the targeted nature of neurofeedback, allowing for a more concentrated and personalized therapy approach.

Designing Personalized Neurofeedback Protocols involves the creation of therapeutic objectives. This stage entails developing a personalized strategy based on the individual's neurophysiological profile and detected dysregulations. The practitioner uses the data from the QEEG mapping and clinical interviews to create a treatment that treats the precise brain patterns causing the client's symptoms. This individualized approach distinguishes neurofeedback therapy from other generic approaches. The protocols may involve targeting certain brainwave frequencies or using neurofeedback approaches tailored to the client's requirements.

Neurofeedback Sessions and Equipment are the practical applications of the designed protocols. The sessions usually involve the client using neurofeedback equipment, which delivers real-time feedback on their brainwave activity. This feedback is frequently sent in the form of visual or aural cues, allowing the user to gain awareness and control over their neural pathways.

The technology used in neurofeedback sessions varies, but it typically involves EEG (Electroencephalography) sensors, amplifiers, and a computer interface. The client's active engagement in these sessions is critical because they learn to adjust their brain activity in response to feedback, gradually improving neural functioning.

Continuous assessment and adjustment are critical components of the neurofeedback process. Regular progress evaluations, such as repeat QEEG mappings, ensure that the intervention remains personalized to the individual's changing needs.

The flexibility in adjusting neurofeedback protocols allows for the accommodation of changes in the client's neurophysiological profile during therapy. This iterative method stresses neurofeedback's dynamic character and its ability to provide individualized and adaptive therapies.

Beyond the technical components, it is necessary to identify the therapeutic bond between the practitioner and the client as an important part of the neurofeedback process. The practitioner's experience and assistance provide a supportive environment, allowing the client to participate and commit to the intervention.

This collaborative relationship improves the overall efficacy of neurofeedback therapy by making the client feel understood, motivated, and empowered along their path of neurophysiological self-regulation.

The Neurofeedback Process represents a paradigm shift in therapeutic interventions, providing a more nuanced and tailored approach to treating neurophysiological dysfunction. From the rigorous Initial Assessment and Client Evaluation to the dynamic Neurofeedback Sessions and Equipment, each aspect contributes to the overall goal of enhancing brain function and increasing mental well-being. As the discipline evolves, continued study and improvement of neurofeedback techniques hold the possibility of broadening its usefulness across a wide range of clinical domains, thereby confirming its status as a key tool in neuropsychological therapies.

CHAPTER 4
CONDITIONS TREATED WITH NEUROFEEDBACK

Neurofeedback therapy has gained popularity as a non-invasive, drug-free way to treat a variety of neurological and psychiatric disorders.

This novel therapy approach uses real-time monitoring of brain activity to improve self-regulation and overall brain function. Attention-deficit/hyperactivity disorder (ADHD) is one of the most common conditions treated with neurofeedback.

ADHD and neurofeedback

ADHD is a neurodevelopmental condition defined by persistent patterns of inattention, hyperactivity, and impulsivity.

Neurofeedback therapy for ADHD tries to adjust and optimize the brain's activity patterns, focusing on the areas responsible for attention and impulse control.

Individuals with ADHD can learn to regulate their brainwaves using operant training, which leads to improved focus, less impulsivity, and improved executive functioning.

Numerous researches has yielded positive results, indicating that neurofeedback can be used as an effective supplement or alternative to standard ADHD therapies.

Moving beyond ADHD, neurofeedback is effective in treating anxiety disorders, providing a unique and customized approach to addressing the complex manifestations of anxiety.

Anxiety disorders and neurofeedback

Anxiety disorders, which include ailments like generalized anxiety disorder (GAD), social anxiety disorder, and panic disorder, are defined by excessive and uncontrollable worry, fear, and trepidation.

Neurofeedback therapy for anxiety tries to change the underlying brain processes that cause heightened arousal and stress responses. By delivering real-time feedback, people can learn to self-regulate their brain activity, resulting in a more balanced and adaptable response to stimuli. Neurofeedback has shown promise in terms of anxiety reduction, emotional regulation, and overall well-being.

Similarly, depression, a common and debilitating mental health issue, has been a focus of neurofeedback intervention.

Depression & Neurofeedback

Depression is characterized by continuous sorrow, pessimism, and a loss of interest in activities. Neurofeedback for depression addresses neural dysregulation associated with mood disorders, with a focus on modifying brainwave patterns related to emotional processing and regulation. Neurofeedback, which trains people to create a more balanced and adaptive brain state, may help to alleviate depression symptoms. According to research in this field, neurofeedback can be an effective component of comprehensive depression treatment strategies, either as a standalone intervention or in concert with other therapy techniques.

Post-Traumatic Stress Disorder (PTSD) is another area where neurofeedback has shown promise as a treatment.

Post-traumatic Stress Disorder (PTSD) and neurofeedback

PTSD is a complex mental health disease that can develop in response to traumatic situations. Neurofeedback therapy for PTSD tries to address the underlying neurological imbalances caused by trauma, focusing on areas of the brain involved in fear processing and emotion control.

Neurofeedback, which trains people to alter their brainwave patterns, may help reduce the hyperarousal and reactivity that are frequent in PTSD. While further research is needed, preliminary findings suggest that neurofeedback can help people with PTSD reduce symptoms and enhance their quality of life.

Neurofeedback expands its application to pain management, providing a non-pharmacological solution to ease suffering.

Neurofeedback and Pain Management

Chronic pain is a complex and frequently difficult condition to manage. Neurofeedback in pain management focuses on how the brain perceives and processes pain signals. Neurofeedback, by addressing neural networks involved in pain perception, aims to improve pain modulation and overall pain experience.

This approach provides a viable alternate or complementary strategy to established pain treatment strategies, perhaps minimizing the need for pharmacological therapies.

While research in this field is still ongoing, preliminary findings indicate that neurofeedback may hold promise for people looking for non-pharmacological choices for chronic pain treatment.

Cognitive enhancement is a specialized use of neurofeedback that caters to people looking to improve their cognitive ability.

Neurofeedback for Cognitive Enhancement.

Cognitive enhancement refers to tactics and interventions designed to improve cognitive processes like memory, attention, and problem-solving. Neurofeedback for cognitive enhancement is based on the idea that certain brainwave patterns are connected with peak cognitive performance.

Neurofeedback aims to improve cognitive capacities by teaching people how to achieve and sustain these patterns.

This application has sparked interest in a variety of situations, including academic and professional settings, as well as individuals who want to maximize their cognitive potential. While the field of cognitive enhancement through neurofeedback is still developing, preliminary research indicates that tailored neurofeedback interventions may contribute to improved cognitive functioning.

Neurofeedback treatment is a versatile and growing approach to treating a variety of neurological and psychiatric problems. Neurofeedback remains an active field of research and therapeutic inquiry, with applications ranging from ADHD to anxiety, depression, PTSD, pain treatment, and cognitive development. As our understanding of the complex relationship between brain function and mental health grows, neurofeedback has the potential to provide tailored and effective interventions for people seeking alternatives or complements to standard therapy approaches.

CHAPTER 5
CASE STUDIES

Neurofeedback Therapy has gained popularity in recent years as a non-invasive and promising treatment for a variety of neurological and psychological problems. In this talk, we will look at three key topics: successful neurofeedback treatment cases, challenges and solutions in neurofeedback therapy, and long-term effects and follow-up.

Successful neurofeedback treatment cases:

Examining successful treatment cases across a wide range of neurological and psychiatric diseases is a critical component of verifying the efficacy of Neurofeedback Therapy. Numerous studies have shown promising results, demonstrating the effectiveness of neurofeedback in treating illnesses such as attention-deficit/hyperactivity disorder (ADHD), anxiety disorders, and even traumatic brain injuries. In the case of ADHD, for example, neurofeedback has shown promise in increasing attention span, decreasing impulsivity, and improving general cognitive performance. Case studies frequently illustrate the customized character of neurofeedback protocols, which adjust treatment to each patient's specific neurophysiological profile. Success stories demonstrate the flexibility of neurofeedback across varied demographics, adding to the expanding body of evidence supporting its usefulness.

Furthermore, neurofeedback has shown potential in treating anxiety disorders, with case studies revealing a decrease in symptoms such as excessive concern, panic attacks, and social anxiety. The neuroplasticity-oriented method of neurofeedback is expected to help reshape maladaptive brain processes associated with anxiety. Neurofeedback has also been effective in treating traumatic brain injuries (TBIs). Case reports show that people suffering from TBIs have improved their cognitive function, emotional management, and quality of life. These outcomes highlight neurofeedback's promise as a diverse therapy method capable of addressing a wide range of neurological and psychological issues.

Challenges and Solutions for Neurofeedback Therapy:

While neurofeedback therapy has shown potential, it does not come without problems. One significant difficulty is the heterogeneity in individual responses to neurofeedback treatments. Age, disease severity, and comorbidities can all have an impact on treatment outcomes. Furthermore, keeping patient interest during the course of neurofeedback therapy can be difficult, especially for those who do not immediately see substantial gains. Adherence to treatment regimens is critical for best results, and addressing issues of motivation and expectations becomes vital.

Another problem is the standardization of neurofeedback protocols. As a relatively new therapeutic method, research is ongoing to develop standardized regimens for various illnesses. Tailoring neurofeedback to individual neurophysiological profiles is a strength, but striking a balance between individualization and developing generalizable protocols is difficult. Researchers and practitioners are actively attempting to refine and standardize protocols to improve result repeatability and promote broader adoption within the medical and psychological sectors.

Technological challenges also arise, notably about the accessibility and affordability of neurofeedback equipment. While progress has been made in making devices more portable and cost-effective, ensuring wider availability remains a challenge. Addressing these problems will necessitate coordinated efforts from researchers, doctors, and technology developers to refine protocols, improve accessibility, and improve overall effectiveness.

Long-Term Effects and Follow-up:

Understanding the long-term consequences of neurofeedback therapy is critical for assessing its ongoing impact on neurological and psychological well-being. While several case studies and short-term trials have shown promising results, longitudinal studies are required to establish the long-term viability of these effects. Research in this area has shown promising results, with multiple studies finding that gains in attention, cognitive function, and emotional regulation continue long after neurofeedback treatment is completed.

Long-term follow-up studies in ADHD populations, for example, suggest that the advantages of neurofeedback may last beyond the active treatment phase. However, the magnitude and duration of these effects can differ between individuals. It is crucial to highlight that the long-term benefits of neurofeedback may be influenced by variables such as the individual's age at the time of treatment, the severity of the ailment, and the presence of any ongoing therapeutic therapies.

Long-term follow-up studies in anxiety disorders reveal that neurofeedback may help to reduce anxiety symptoms over the long term. These findings suggest that neurofeedback-induced neuroplastic alterations may have long-term consequences on brain circuits responsible for emotional control. Understanding the processes underlying these long-term consequences is a major focus of current study in the subject.

When investigating long-term impacts, it is critical to consider the possibility of relapse or worsening of symptoms.

Longitudinal studies that follow individuals over time can provide information on the factors that may influence the maintenance or decrease of treatment gains. Identifying determinants of sustained improvement is critical for fine-tuning treatment regimens and maximizing long-term outcomes.

The study of successful neurofeedback treatment cases, problems, and solutions, as well as long-term impacts and follow-up, provides a thorough picture of the current state of neurofeedback therapy. While success stories demonstrate its promise in a variety of situations, problems highlight the need for continual improvement and standardization.

Long-term research provides vital insights about neurofeedback's long-term influence, influencing the future course of this innovative treatment strategy.

CHAPTER 6

INTEGRATING NEUROFEEDBACK AND OTHER THERAPIES

The combination of neurofeedback therapy with complementary therapies is a modern approach to comprehensive mental health care. Complementary therapies, which include a variety of modalities such as mindfulness meditation, yoga, and acupuncture, are essential in creating a holistic healing environment. Neurofeedback, which focuses on controlling brain activity, complements existing treatments by targeting the underlying neurological pathways that contribute to mental health illnesses. For example, integrating neurofeedback and mindfulness practices can improve self-regulation abilities while also developing a more resilient and adaptive mind-body link. This integrative method takes advantage of the synergies between neurofeedback and complementary therapies, offering clients a complex and tailored treatment plan that addresses both cognitive and emotional elements of their well-being.

In conjunction with complementary therapies, the combination of neurofeedback and medicine constitutes a diverse approach to mental health therapy. Medication is frequently administered to treat symptoms of psychiatric diseases by addressing neurotransmitter imbalances in the brain. In contrast, neurofeedback uses operant conditioning to regulate brain activity. Combining these techniques has the potential to improve treatment outcomes because neurofeedback can help optimize drug effects. For example, neurofeedback could be used to target specific brain regions related to pharmaceutical response, potentially lowering dosage or reducing adverse effects. However, integrating neurofeedback with medication requires careful consideration of individual characteristics, response patterns, and potential contraindications, emphasizing the need for tailored treatment programs to maximize therapeutic effects.

Neurofeedback combined with psychotherapy is a dynamic and promising approach to mental health treatment. Psychotherapy, based on diverse theoretical frameworks such as cognitive-behavioral therapy (CBT) or psychodynamic therapy, tackles the psychological and emotional components of mental health illnesses. In contrast, neurofeedback works on a neurobiological level, focusing on dysregulated brain activity. Integrating these modalities can improve the overall efficacy of mental health treatment by addressing both cognitive and emotional elements simultaneously. Neurofeedback, for example, can be used to reinforce favorable cognitive-behavioral patterns or to help people regulate their emotions during psychotherapy sessions. This integration allows for a more complete view of the individual by incorporating both psychological and neurobiological elements into the diagnostic and therapy process. However, successful integration requires collaboration between neurofeedback practitioners and psychotherapists, with an emphasis on multidisciplinary communication and agreed on treatment goals.

The combination of neurofeedback therapy, complementary therapies, medication, and psychotherapy emphasizes the necessity of a multifaceted and tailored treatment approach. While each modality has unique strengths and mechanisms of action, their synergistic synthesis provides a more comprehensive view of mental health. This integrated approach highlights the subtle interplay of cognitive, emotional, and neurological processes, allowing for a more nuanced understanding of individual needs and therapies that are tailored accordingly. As the field evolves, further study and collaboration among other therapeutic disciplines will be critical in improving and expanding the efficacy of integrated neurofeedback therapy.

CHAPTER 7
ETHICAL AND PROFESSIONAL CONSIDERATIONS

Neurofeedback treatment is a rapidly growing area that uses real-time displays of brain activity to teach self-regulation of brain function. As the field evolves, it is critical to address the ethical and professional considerations that underpin neurofeedback practice. This section will go over three important topics: Ethical Guidelines for Neurofeedback Practitioners, Informed

Consent and Client Rights, and Continuous Professional Development in Neurofeedback.

Ethical guidelines for neurofeedback practitioners:

Neurofeedback practitioners play an important role in guiding people through the process of self-regulating their brain function. As with any therapy intervention, following ethical norms is critical to ensuring the client's well-being and maintaining the profession's integrity. One of the most important ethical considerations in neurofeedback therapy is the requirement for practitioners to maintain confidentiality. The sensitive nature of the information acquired during neurofeedback sessions emphasizes the need to protect clients' privacy. Practitioners must set clear boundaries with clients and discuss the constraints of confidentiality to create trust in the therapeutic relationship.

Additionally, neurofeedback practitioners must be attentive in getting informed permission from clients before beginning therapy.

Informed consent entails giving clients detailed information on the nature of neurofeedback, potential risks and benefits, alternative treatment choices, and the practitioner's credentials. This procedure gives clients the ability to make educated decisions regarding their participation in neurofeedback therapy, supporting autonomy and respect for personal choice. Practitioners should also be open about the limitations of neurofeedback and manage client expectations realistically.

Furthermore, ethical neurofeedback practitioners follow the idea of competence. Maintaining a high level of professional competency requires continual education, training, and supervision.

As the area of neurofeedback advances, practitioners must keep up with the newest research, methodologies, and ethical standards. Continuous professional development is required to guarantee that practitioners can provide effective and evidence-based therapies while maintaining the highest ethical standards.

The ethical criteria for neurofeedback practitioners include protecting confidentiality, gaining informed permission, and maintaining competence. T hese principles serve as the foundation for a professional and ethical approach that promotes client well-being and helps to build the credibility of the neurofeedback discipline.

Informed Consent and Client Rights:

Informed consent is a crucial ethical premise in neurofeedback therapy that emphasizes autonomy and respect for the client's rights. Before beginning therapy, neurofeedback practitioners must get informed permission from clients to ensure that they understand the nature of the intervention, the risks and benefits, and their rights in the therapeutic process. The process of getting informed permission is more than just a formality; it is an ongoing discourse that allows clients to make educated decisions regarding their involvement in neurofeedback therapy.

One important aspect of informed consent in neurofeedback is to ensure that clients understand the intervention's goals and objectives. Clients should be educated on the exact neurofeedback protocols that will be utilized, the anticipated duration of the therapy, and the potential outcomes.

This honesty helps to control client expectations and promotes a collaborative therapy partnership based on mutual understanding.

Furthermore, practitioners must explain the potential dangers and benefits of neurofeedback therapy. While neurofeedback is generally thought to be safe, clients are entitled to be informed of any potential side effects or unpleasant responses. This information allows clients to assess the possible benefits of neurofeedback against the dangers involved and make decisions that are consistent with their values and interests.

Respecting clients' rights is an essential component of ethical neurofeedback practice. Practitioners must ensure that clients understand their right to withdraw from therapy at any moment without fear of pressure or punishment. This allows clients to take an active role in their treatment, contributing to a therapeutic atmosphere based on trust and collaboration.

The ethical practice of neurofeedback therapy requires informed consent and respect for client rights. Practitioners can lay the groundwork for a therapeutic partnership that improves the success of neurofeedback interventions by emphasizing autonomy, transparency, and respect for their clients' decisions.

Continuing Professional Development in Neurofeedback:

Continuous professional development (CPD) is an essential component of ethical and effective neurofeedback practice. Because neuroscience and neurofeedback technologies are continually improving, practitioners must continue their education, training, and supervision to maintain competency and deliver high-quality care to clients. This section investigates the significance of CPD in neurofeedback and the many methods by which practitioners can improve their knowledge and abilities.

One of the key reasons for participating in ongoing professional development is to stay current on the newest advances in neurofeedback research and practice. The field is dynamic, with new studies and technology developing regularly. Practitioners who commit to continuous professional development can include evidence-based interventions in their practice, ensuring that clients receive the most up-to-date and effective neurofeedback protocols.

Furthermore, CPD allows neurofeedback practitioners to broaden their professional skills and diversify their treatment approaches. Practitioners can obtain experience in specialized areas of neurofeedback by attending workshops, conferences, and advanced training programs, such as treating specific clinical disorders or employing sophisticated neuroimaging techniques.

This enhanced understanding improves practitioners' capacity to tailor neurofeedback therapies to the specific needs of individual clients.

Supervision is another important aspect of CPD in neurofeedback. Regular supervision allows practitioners to discuss difficult situations, receive feedback on their therapeutic skills, and maintain ethical and professional standards. Supervision also promotes a sense of community among practitioners, allowing for peer support and collaboration.

Furthermore, participating in CPD shows a commitment to ethical and professional development. Clients can be confident that practitioners who invest in continuing education are committed to giving the best possible service and remaining current on the newest advances in the profession. This dedication to perfection boosts the legitimacy of neurofeedback as a therapeutic modality and helps to promote the profession.

Continuous professional development is required for neurofeedback practitioners to maintain competence, keep up with industry innovations, and improve their clinical abilities. By focusing on continuous education, training, and supervision, practitioners can contribute to the ethical and effective practice of neurofeedback therapy while also supporting professional growth and development.

CHAPTER 8
FUTURE TRENDS IN NEUROFEEDBACK

Advancements in neurofeedback technology:

The discipline of neurofeedback therapy has seen tremendous technological breakthroughs, which have transformed how brain activity is monitored and managed. One of the most significant technological advances has been the creation of more advanced EEG (electroencephalogram) devices. Modern EEG technology now enables for finer resolution and more exact monitoring of brainwave patterns, giving physicians detailed information regarding neural activity. These developments help to optimize neurofeedback procedures, making them more targeted and effective.

Another significant advancement in neurofeedback technology is the incorporation of real-time functional magnetic resonance imaging (fMRI) feedback. This breakthrough enables therapists to detect and study changes in brain activity with unprecedented precision. Real-time fMRI neurofeedback enables a more comprehensive understanding of the brain's response to diverse stimuli and interventions, allowing for tailored and adaptable neurofeedback regimens. The combination of EEG and fMRI technology provides new opportunities for treating complicated neurological and psychological problems by targeting both structural and functional components of the brain.

Furthermore, wearable neurofeedback devices have become more popular, allowing people to practice neurofeedback outside of therapeutic settings.

These portable gadgets, which commonly take the form of headsets or headbands, allow users to monitor and control their brain activity in real-time. The accessibility of neurofeedback via wearable technology broadens the scope of this therapeutic technique, allowing people to actively participate in their mental health. As technology advances, we should expect additional miniaturization and enhancements to these devices, making neurofeedback more accessible and convenient for users.

Emerging Research & Discovery:

The field of neurofeedback therapy is always changing, thanks to ongoing research that advances our understanding of the brain's complex processes. Emerging studies investigate new applications and improve old protocols, offering light on the mechanisms that underpin neurofeedback's therapeutic effects. Neuroscientists are studying the intricacies of brain plasticity, including how neurofeedback produces long-term changes in neural networks and connectivity.

Recent studies have concentrated on the combination of neurofeedback with other therapeutic modalities, such as cognitive-behavioral therapy (CBT) and pharmaceutical therapies. Combining neurofeedback with known treatments has the potential to improve overall therapy outcomes, particularly in the case of complicated mental health conditions. Studies on the synergistic effects of neurofeedback and psychopharmacology, for example, seek to determine the best combinations for more personalized and effective treatment strategies.

Furthermore, neurofeedback research is broadening to include a wider range of neurological and psychiatric disorders. While neurofeedback was initially studied for illnesses such as ADHD and anxiety, current research has looked into its efficacy in treating depression, post-traumatic stress disorder (PTSD), and neurodevelopmental disorders. The comprehensive understanding gained from these studies contributes to the continual refining of neurofeedback procedures and broadens their potential applications.

Individual disparities in treatment outcomes are also being investigated through neurofeedback research. Age, gender, and genetic predispositions are being studied to see how these affect responses to neurofeedback. This individualized method seeks to adjust neurofeedback interventions to each individual's unique neurobiology, hence increasing the therapy's effectiveness. As research in this field improves, we should expect more precise and personalized neurofeedback methods.

Potential Applications and Expansions:

Neurofeedback therapy has far-reaching potential applications, with academics and doctors investigating a wide range of areas where brain regulation can improve health and well-being. One major growth is the use of neurofeedback to improve cognitive performance and optimize brain function in healthy people. Cognitive improvement neurofeedback programs are designed to increase attention, memory, and executive functions in persons seeking optimal cognitive performance in academic, professional, or artistic endeavors.

Neurofeedback is also being investigated as an additional treatment in rehabilitation settings. According to research, it could help people recover from traumatic brain injuries, strokes, or neurodegenerative illnesses. The versatility of neurofeedback protocols enables therapists to customize therapies to address specific cognitive deficiencies and encourage neuroplasticity during the rehabilitation process. Integrating neurofeedback into established rehabilitation procedures creates new opportunities for improving recovery results.

Furthermore, the use of neurofeedback is expanding into sports psychology, where it is utilized to improve athletes' mental resilience, attention, and performance. Neurofeedback training can help athletes improve their performance and learn new skills more quickly. As this application grows in popularity, we may anticipate the creation of specialized neurofeedback protocols adapted to the specific cognitive demands of particular sports.

In the field of mental health, neurofeedback is broadening its application to treat a wider range of diseases. Studies are being conducted to determine its effectiveness in treating illnesses such as obsessive-compulsive disorder (OCD), bipolar disorder, and eating disorders. Neurofeedback's non-invasive nature makes it an appealing choice for people who are hesitant to try pharmacological therapies or traditional psychotherapy.

CONCLUSION

Neurofeedback therapy is at the forefront of novel approaches to mental health and cognitive well-being. Neurofeedback has evolved into a diverse and promising treatment modality as technology advances and new research and discoveries emerge.

The advancement of neurofeedback technology, which includes advanced EEG equipment, real-time fMRI feedback, and wearable devices, demonstrates the commitment to refining and broadening the scope of this therapeutic method.

The current research in neurofeedback not only advances our understanding of the underlying mechanisms, but also broadens the range of potential applications.

The investigation of neurofeedback in conjunction with other treatment modalities, as well as its application to a wide range of domains such as rehabilitation, sports psychology, and cognitive enhancement, demonstrate the intervention's adaptability and versatility. Furthermore, the emphasis on individualized treatment approaches, taking into account aspects such as age, gender, and genetic predispositions, ushers in a more personalized and effective era of neurofeedback therapy.

As neurofeedback therapy evolves, its potential to treat a wide range of neurological and mental problems becomes more apparent. Neurofeedback's non-invasive nature, combined with its capacity to generate long-term alterations in brain networks, makes it a useful addition to the therapeutic landscape. Neurofeedback is becoming more accessible, whether used in clinical settings or via portable wearable devices, allowing people to actively participate in their mental health and well-being.

Looking ahead, the future of neurofeedback therapy looks promising, with further technological advancements, ongoing innovative research, and an ever-expanding range of applications. Neurofeedback is evolving into a dynamic and disruptive discipline at the convergence of neuroscience, technology, and personalized medicine, with significant contributions to mental health care and cognitive optimization on the horizon.

www.ingramcontent.com/pod-product-compliance
Lightning Source LLC
Chambersburg PA
CBHW070813290526
45795CB00002B/706